Natural Pain Relief with Foods, Herbs & Essential Oils

74 Simple Remedies to Get Relief

Kathy Wyatt

© 2017

The information herein is offered for informational purposes solely, and is universal as so. The presentation of the information is without contract or any type of guarantee assurance.
The trademarks that are used are without any consent, and the publication of the trademark is without permission or backing by the trademark owner. All trademarks and brands within this book are for clarifying purposes only and are the owned by the owners themselves, not affiliated with this document.

Any advice given in this book is for informational purposes only and is not considered to cure, treat, or prevent any disease. Should you need medical attention, please visit your doctor.

Table of Contents

Introduction

Pain is something that we all know far too well. It's a part of living that cannot be avoided, and yet you don't have to deal with it. There are many methods out there to deal with pain, and one of the most common is getting a prescription from your doctor. This often leads to addiction and dependence, but what if I told you there was a healthier alternative that worked just as well? There are many natural ways that you can get rid of pain. There is no reason to rely on manufactured pills. Even if you can get pain killers from your doctor, there is a stigma that comes with taking them that many people want to avoid. Natural remedies are better in the long term, especially if you are dealing with chronic pain.

Chapter 1: 10 Reasons to Go Natural

Herbal and natural remedies have been available for centuries. Many people that are used to taking care of a busy home are skilled in basic remedies. Though, this common knowledge is slowly disappearing as it's easier and easier to send for a doctor or go to see one. Many people even believe that herbal remedies are just new age remedies, and this simply isn't true. Everyone has their own reasons for going natural, but some of these are some universal reasons that almost everyone can agree on.

Less Side Effects

One of the most common reasons is that people are tired of dealing with the side effects that comes with mainstream medication. Natural medication does not have the same side effects as pharmaceuticals. Unless you're having a reaction, there shouldn't be any side effects at all. There's no warning labels telling you that you'll likely become addicted or shouldn't drive while taking it.

Your Body Takes to It

Your body makes use of anything that you put into it. However, your body is more prone to handling a natural remedy better than pharmaceuticals. For many people the herbal remedy lasts longer, and it just leaves you with an overall better feeling. This helps you to be more efficient, and it's a large reason why many people take herbal remedies for chronic pain. You have to think about what it's doing to your body long term, and herbal remedies are simply the better option.

There's No Middle Man

Many medications on the market have come a long ways from their natural counterpart, but they did actually come from something natural. This is especially true when you're dealing with pain killers. There's no reason to go to the source. No one likes having to go through one channel and then the next just to get their pain relief. It shouldn't be mentally painful to take care of your body, and by taking your pain relief in your own hands, you're helping to cut down on this mentally fatiguing activity.

They are Safer

Pharmaceutical companies don't always test products all the way through, which can put you at risk. It's expensive when they're trying to develop new medication, so they're likely to cut corners to try to get their product on the market sooner. However, always keep in mind that you shouldn't just come off of medication you really need. There are conditions that are better treated by using pharmaceutical medications, but pain is usually not one of them. Though, there is a chance that herbal remedies could interact with over the counter medication, this doesn't happen often. As long as you consult an expert before adding various herbal remedies, over the counter medications and pharmaceuticals, it's safe to use herbal remedies for a natural pain relief.

It Costs Less

One of the main reasons that many people choose to go with a natural remedy for pain is because it costs less than pain killers, especially if you're in the US. Many people are stuck trying to decide between getting their medication, getting food or paying a bill. Not all insurances will cover all medications, and there isn't always a generic option. Natural remedies simply cost less, and if you grow your own herbs, they can cost even less.

Natural Remedies Have History

Many people feel assured that the natural method will work because they have a history of being used. Natural pain relief can be tracked across human history, and you can find proof of it working. There is documentation about herbal medications throughout time that can be researched and referenced. Many pharmaceutical medications have not been around nearly as long.

They Are Just as Effective

Many people worry that natural remedies aren't as potent, but you'll soon find out that this just isn't true. They're just as effective as pharmaceuticals. Some natural remedies will even work better and last longer. It's normal to think that the newest thing is the best, but this just isn't true. The older remedies have withstood the test of time. These are tried and true remedies that are guaranteed to work.

Easier on the Planet

You should also think about the footprint that you're leaving behind. When you're using a product that has been manufactured, then it will leave a footprint. Pharmaceuticals have a negative impact on the planet. Natural remedies are earth friendly, and they're sustainable alternatives. You can even grow many of these herbal remedies to help cut down on costs.

Providing For Yourself

Natural pain relief allows you to be self-sufficient, meaning you can provide for yourself. There's a bit of pride that comes with self-sufficiency and knowing that you're handling your pain on your own. Though, it's the simple fact that you can choose to take herbal medicine over the alternatives. It is a decision that you'll need to make for yourself.

Chapter 2: Herbal Remedies

When people think natural pain relief they usually think about herbs first. This is one method to handle pain relief naturally, and it can be one of the most effective and well used methods out there. There are many herbal remedies that work for different types of pain. You can treat headaches, toothaches, and even chronic pain with various herbal remedies. There are some herbal remedies that derive from food, and other herbal remedies actually come from plants. Just keep in mind that certain remedies work differently depending on your own body and how they react to certain medications.

There is always a little bit of trial
and error when trying to figure out
herbal remedy or medication will
work best for you. Just don't panic
if something that you try first
doesn't work. Take a deep breath
and try to move onto another
remedy that might work better for
you. It's best if you start by
keeping a diary or journal of some
type, documenting what recipes do
and do not work for you and your
family.
With herbal remedies you'll be able
to try different things without the
worry of side effects. This gives
you more control. Just remember
to never use any herbal remedies
without consulting a doctor first.
There are many over the counter
medications that can react to these
remedies as well, so it's important
to get a professional opinion before
adding something into your
routine.

Kava Kava

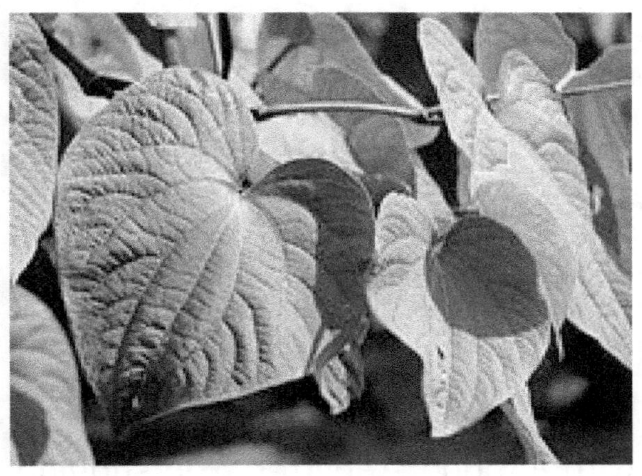

Kava kava isn't a mainstream herb for pain, but it can certainly help with various types of pain that you might be suffering from. However, when you take kava kava you'll need to be careful what you mix it with. Many supplements will work fine with other medications, but kava kava is something you need to be more careful with. Do not take kava kava if you are on medications for mental illness. It often works out badly if you pair it with a mood stabilizer. You should also be aware of your alcohol consumption if you're take kava kava because it can turn into a sedative.

You should not take kava kava if you are operating heavy machinery or doing a lot of driving. It can cause hair and skin discoloration and some people even have allergic reactions. Always talk to a doctor before just adding kava kava, but you should talk to a doctor no matter what supplement that you're adding. Kava kava can help with migraines, chronic pain disorders, sleep, anxiety, and it can act as a muscle relaxant. If you struggle with chronic pain, you'll want to consider taking kava kava despite the added precautions.

Feverfew

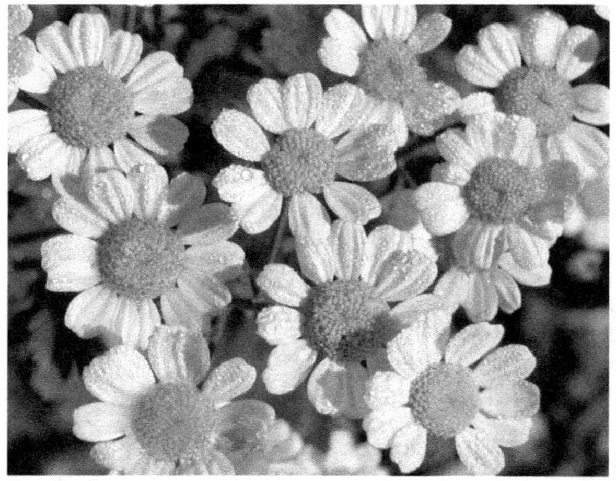

This is a plant that comes from Asia and has been used since ancient times. It's popular because it helps with pain and spread all over the world. There are a few other names for feverfew including Midsummer Daisy, Bachelor's Button, Featherfoil, Featherfew and Matricaria. If you can't find feverfew in your area, then ask a local garden center or club to help you figure out what the title is where you are.

Of course, you can always search the internet as well. Feverfew is common for helping with migraines and headaches. It can also help with cramps from your period and arthritis. It can help to lower fevers as well, and it can even help with stiffness that comes with a bad fever. Feverfew can be used to help with an upset stomach, toothaches and even earaches. You can easily see why this versatile herb spread across the world.

Some people believe that it even helps with tinnitus and psoriasis. You use the leaves of feverfew once they're dried to make a medication. However, you can use fresh leaves as well. It's best if you take it orally. You can crush the leaves in a capsule to make it easier. Though, if you're using feverfew for a toothache, then you'll want to place a leaf directly over the gum or tooth that is causing you the pain. You may be wondering why feverfew works, and it's hard to pinpoint the exact why. It does have a compound known as parthenolide, which is what the body uses to help ease pain and the symptoms that it causes.

Ginseng

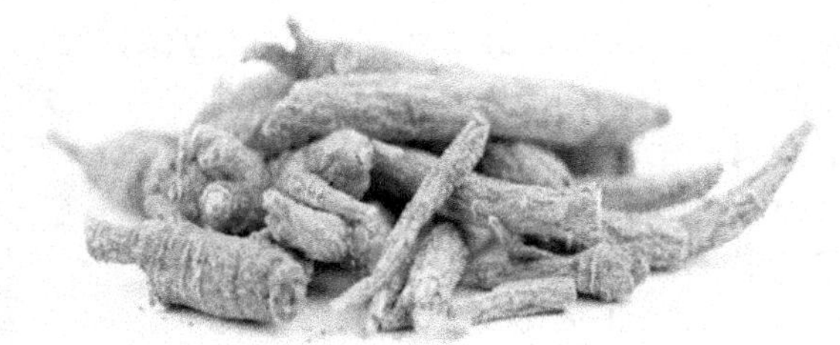

This is another great remedy for pain if you're suffering chronically. Ginseng is great if you are suffering from Fibromyalgia, which can help to give you daily relief. Of course, there are other names for ginseng. It can often be called Ginseng Japonais, Ginseng Blanc de Coree, and Chinese Red Ginseng. Ginseng is from Asian regions, such as Siberia, Korea and China.

You'll see it all over the world now due to its popularity. There is a variety such as Panax Ginseng which is the best variety if you're looking for pain control. This herb also helps with inflammation, controlling infections, COPD, infections of lung disease, pain associated with cancer, memory issues, multiple sclerosis, and even cystic fibrosis. Ginseng is also used in makeups as well as flavoring for food.

Birch Leaf

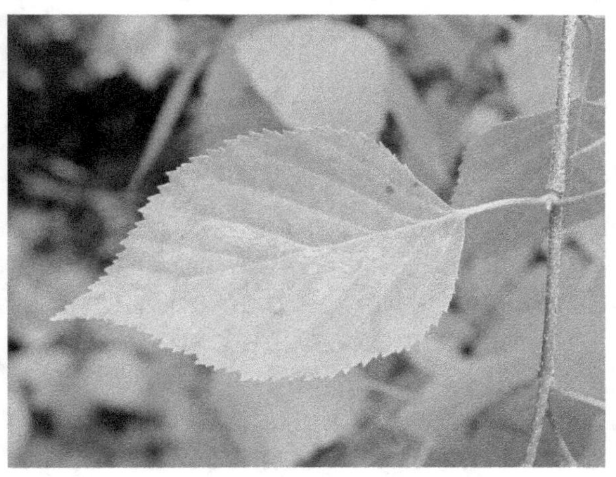

Birch leaf will work much like cortisone which is a prescription drug. It can help with autoimmune disorders, arthritis and more. You'll find a chemical compound called methyl salicylate, which is similar to salicylic acid, which is used in aspirin. It is analgesic, astringent, antifungal, antispasmodic, and it detoxifies you. It's also a diuretic and reduces oxidative damage to your skin, which can help with wrinkles too! It helps to enhance circulation which can cut down on pain too. You can use this as an extract or as an oil, and some people will even use it as a tea.

White Willow Bark

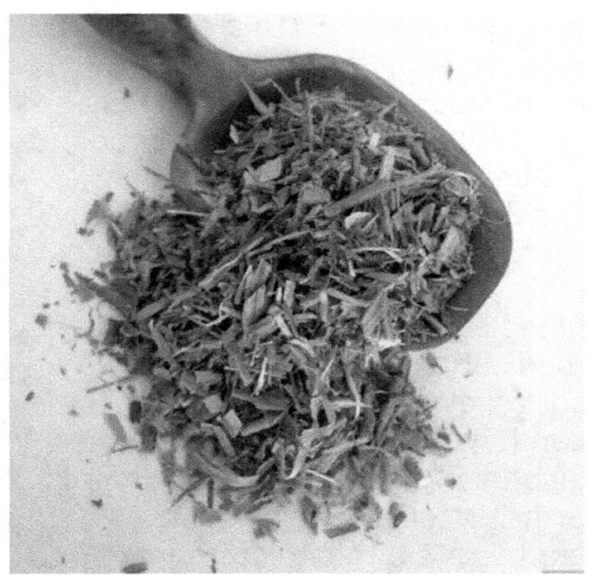

You'll find that white willow bark is a great way to help with pain, and it has salicin in it. This converts to salicylic acid, and it will help to lower your prostaglandin levels which is a hormone like compound which can cause inflammation, aches and pain. The best part is that white willow bark won't upset your stomach or cause internal bleeding, but over the counter medication that uses similar way sot relieve pain, such as aspirin, can have those effects. You can also use this herb for muscle pains, arthritis, or even menstrual cramps. The most common way to use white willow bark is in tea form, but some people will use a tincture or extract as well. It can help after hip or knee surgery too as it reduces inflammation and helps to promote blood flow.

Devil's Claw

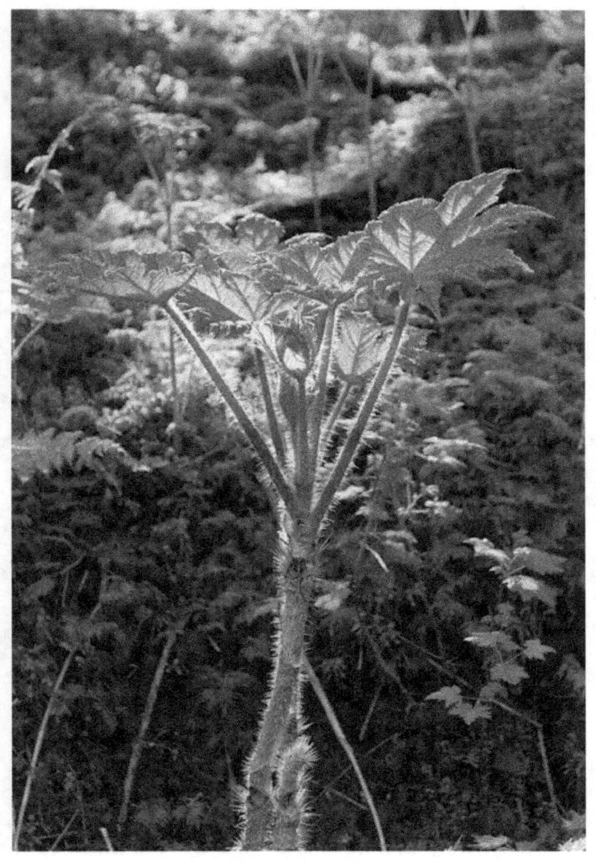

Many people try to avoid this herb simply because of the name, but don't let that scare you away. It has other names such as Grapple Plant, Racine de Windhoek, Garra del Diablo, and Harpagophytum procumbens. Devil's Claw is just the most common name, and it can be the easiest way to find this wonderful herb. It comes from Africa, and when it flowers it has fruit that has hooks all over it. The hooks allow for the fruit to protect itself and spread. The hooks will latch onto animals which spread the seeds all over.

The flower isn't used in herbal remedies, but the root can help to block out pain. It's used to ease the pain of childbirth, gout and arthritis most commonly. It can help with pain that is a result from kidney and bladder issues, burns and back pain. It is also best to take Devil's Claw orally. You can use it topically for some pain such as burns or bug bites. You won't find much modern research on Devil's Claw, and so you should probably not take Devil's Claw if you are pregnant.

Always check with your regular doctor or a homeopathic doctor before you take an herbal remedy when you're expecting a child. Devil's Claw works because it attacks the inflammation that causes pain. You'll see swelling go down, and therefore pain will begin to lessen. If you use it along with heat or ice, you'll notice results even faster.

Aquamin

This comes from red seaweed, and it's a powerful pain reducer. You'll often find this in a pill format, as it's powdered and sold. It'll help with stiffness, and it diminishes inflammation. It will also help to build up bone since its rich in magnesium and calcium. This is better for long term and chronic pain that has to deal with your muscles.

St. John's Wort

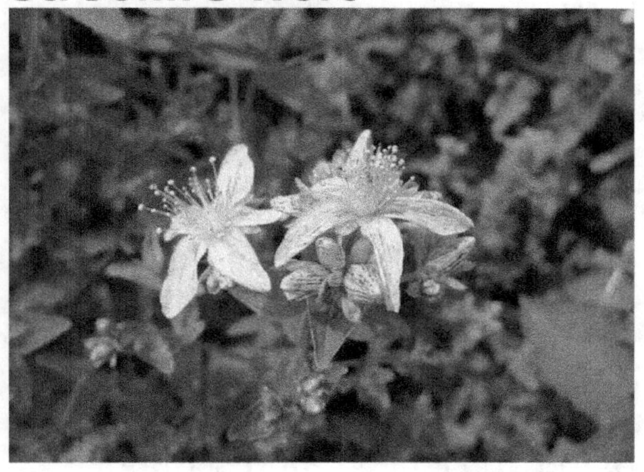

This pain reliever can also help with depression. St. John's Wort is extremely versatile and can help with ADHD, OCD, nerve pain, joint pain, post op pain, Anxiety, HIV and general pain. It's best to take in capsules, but some people prefer to take it in tincture form. You can usually get St. John's Wort over the counter and cheaply. Though, it's worth noting that in some countries in the European Union you'll need a prescription including Ireland. If you're in the US, you should have no issue finding St. John's Wort. The Mayo Clinic has extensively studied and recommends St. John's wort for pain as well as other issues. It is an affordable remedy that is easy to take.

Skullcap

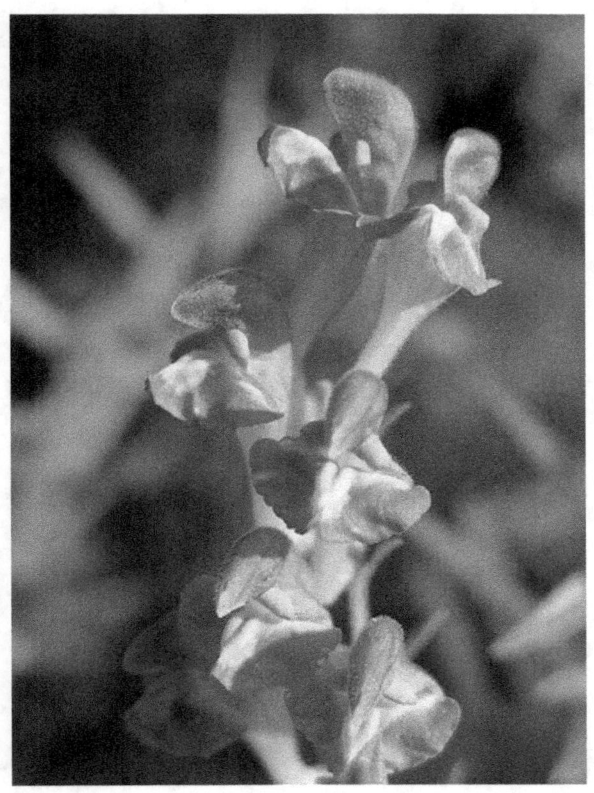

Skullcap is known as a powerful medicinal herb, and it's great when dealing with stress related headaches. Of course, it's also another anti-inflammatory. If you suffer from chronic fatigue syndrome, you may notice a reduction in your pain when using skullcap. You'll want to take this in its supplement form to be safe on dosage.

Acacia

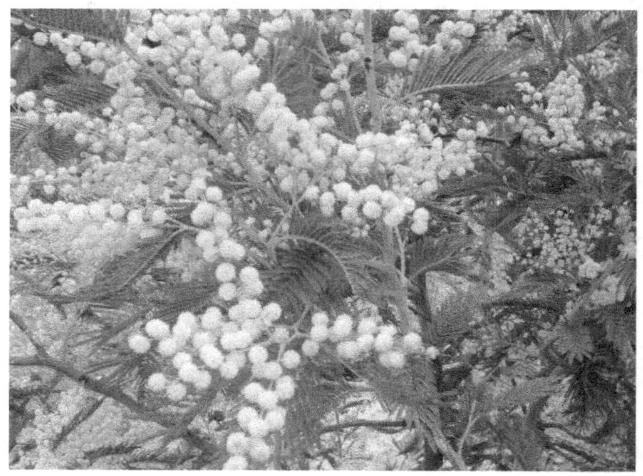

This is a fruit that's native to South Africa, but the bark of that tree is what fights back pain. It can also help to treat bacterial infections, stomach pains and problems, and high blood pressure. You may find a supplement that has acacia blended with boswellia and skullcap for the best results. Just remember to stay with the recommended dosage.

Valerian Root

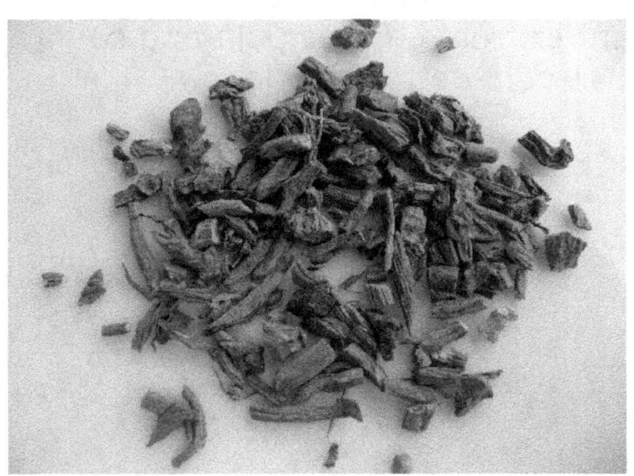

It is known as common valerian,
All-Heal, Garden Heliotrope, and
Herbe aux Coupures. This is
commonly used for people that are
having trouble sleeping, but the
powdered root which is most often
taken in capsules is good at
treating pain. It helps with sleep,
period pains, hot flashes, anxiety
and joint pain. Valerian is still
being studied, but it acts as a
natural sedative. You'll often end
up feeling sleepy when you take it,
but it'll also help to stimulate
nerves that can help with your
pain. This is better for people who
suffer from chronic pain and could
use help getting to sleep.

Aloe Vera

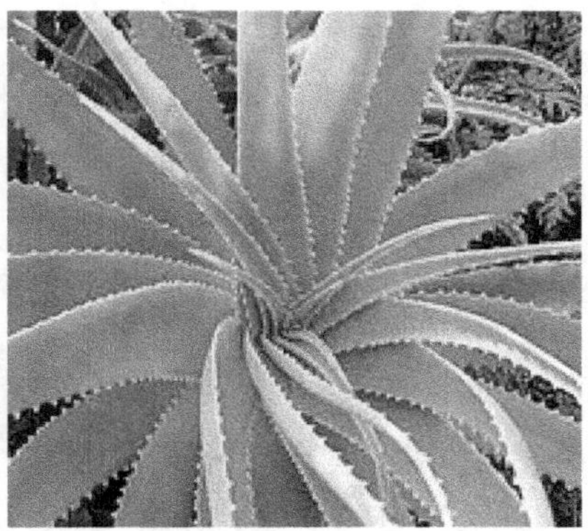

This is known as a remedy for arthritis, and it's a common herb used in the US today. It has powerful anti-inflammatory properties. It also contains vitamin B, C, E and A. it can help to soothe gastrointestinal pain too, and it can help with mouth ulcers. It can be used topically for cold sores, scrapes, burns, cuts and even sunburns. You can drink aloe vera juice or apply it topically for instant relief.

Arnica

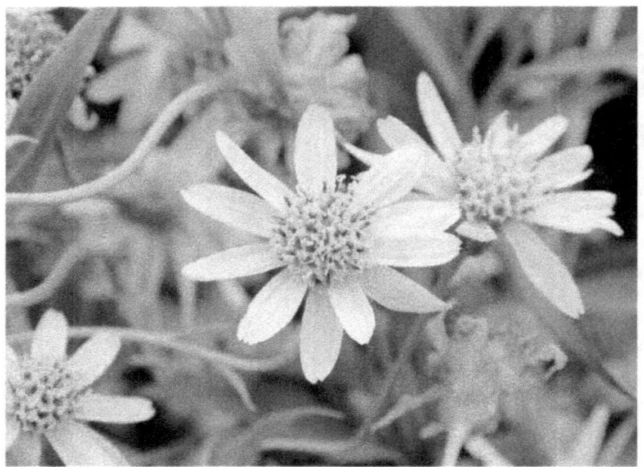

This herb is best if applied topically, and it'll help to relieve sprains, reduce inflammation, and relieve muscle aches. It can help with brushing and helps to heal wounds when applied topically in a salve too. You should not use arnica orally unless it's diluted in a homeopathic solution otherwise you'll have severe side effects. It's best to use arnica topically in salves.

Chamomile

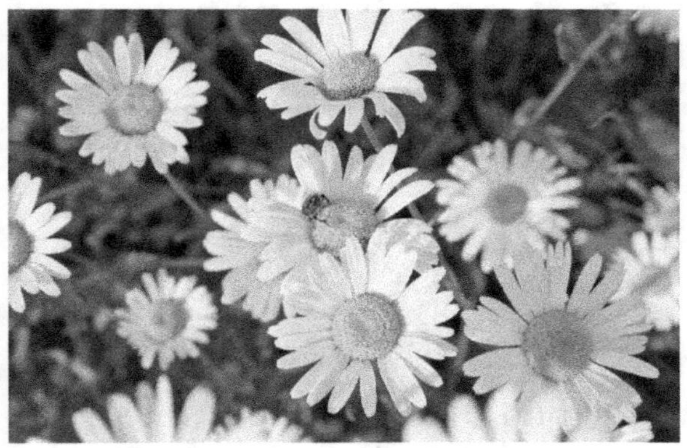

Most people known chamomile from chamomile tea, which many people use as a sleep aid. It can be great if you're lacking sleep due to your chronic pain, but it has a history of being used for hay fever, muscle spasms, menstrual disorders, diaper rash, skin infections, gastrointestinal disorders, inflammation and rheumatic pain too. It's common to take chamomile in tea form to help with pain, but you can also use it topically in a salve.

Neem

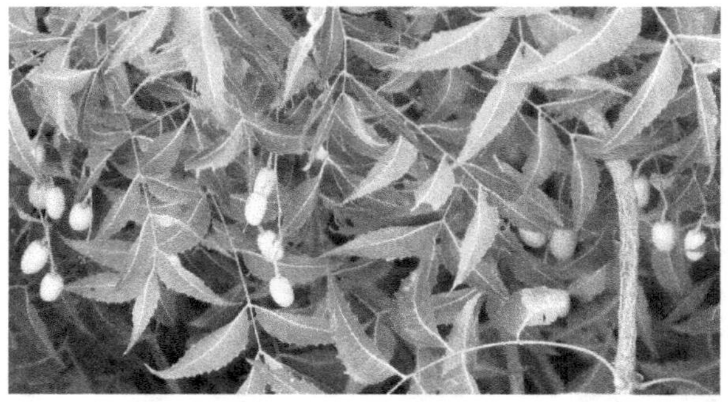

You'll find that most people use neem oil instead of neem because it's easier to get ahold of. However, you'll want to always dilute neem oil in a carrier oil if you use it instead of the herbal form. It's a potent analgesic, which will provide almost instant relief from pain and itching when you apply it topically. It can help to heal cold sores too, and it's commonly used for an upset stomach and muscle pain.

Slippery Elm

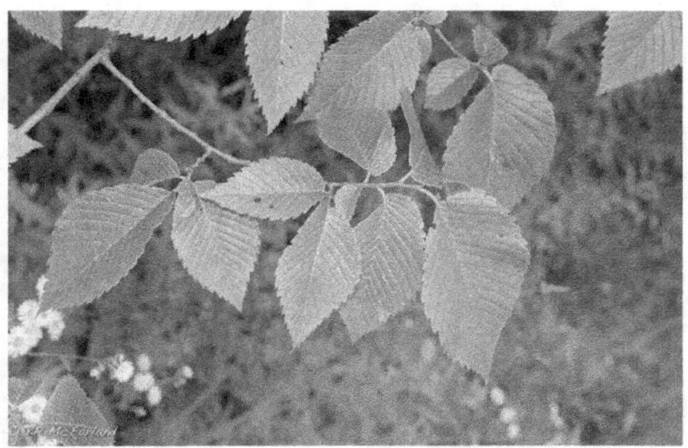

The inner bark is used of the North American elm, known as slippery elm. It's applied directly to the skin, but it can used orally as well in order to relieve sore throats, toothaches, coughs, stomach problems and even diarrhea. When used topically it will help with muscle pain.

Cat's Claw

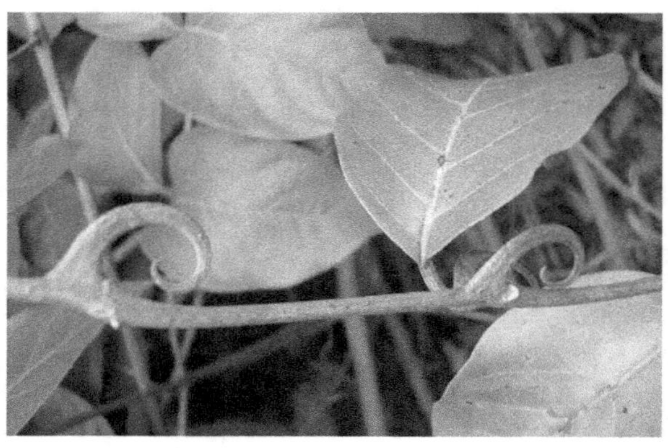

Don't get this mistaken for devil's claw. Cat's claw is from the Amazon rainforest, and it's a woody vine. You'll commonly find it in South America, and it's known as an anti-inflammatory. However, it also stops your body from producing prostaglandin, which is a hormone which contributes to both pain and inflammation. Just make sure to stick to the suggested dosage if you want to avoid diarrhea. When you buy it as a supplement, it'll be easier to determine dosage. If you are buying the powder, then ask your doctor how much you should be taking.

Dandelion

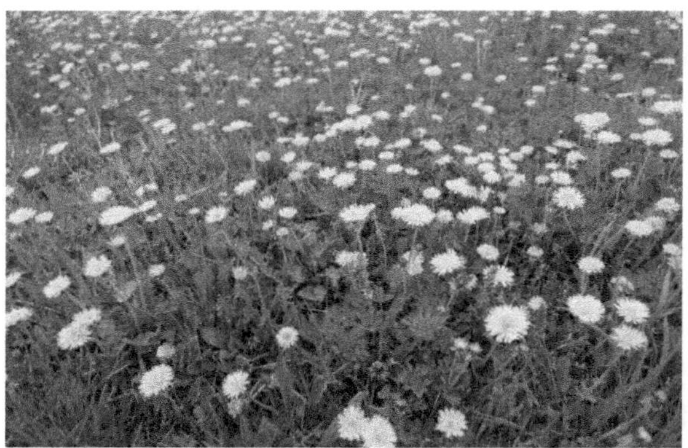

The common flower that you often find growing in your back yard can actually help with joint pain! It's most commonly used in a salve, which you'll find a recipe included later in this book. Just make sure that you don't use dandelion unless you know that it has not been sprayed with pesticides. Always rinse dandelion off before using it, or you can buy it already dried.

Boswellia

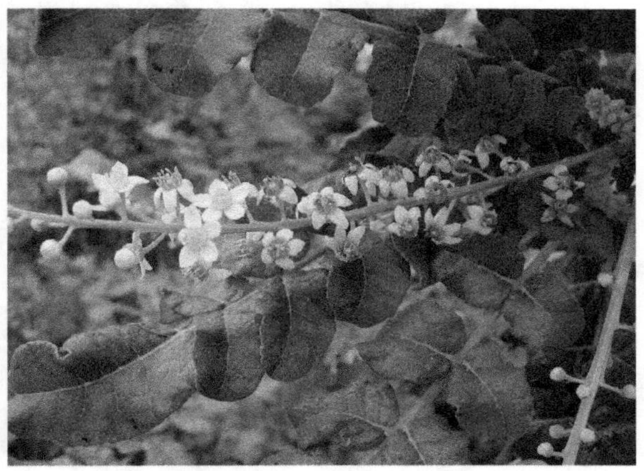

This is another herb that can help you to ease pain, especially muscle pain. It reduces inflammation and stops pain at the source, but it's more common used topically. However, you can buy it in supplement form.

Eucalyptus

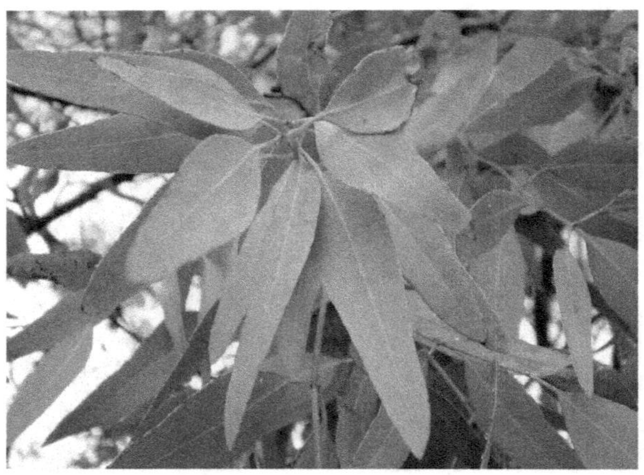

When many people think of eucalyptus, they usually think of cold and flu relief. It is effective for this, but it can be applied topically to alleviate back pain as well. It'll alleviate it in the same way that ice would, using a cooling sensation. Eucalyptus has a substance that's called tanis, and it reduces pain and reduces inflammation at the same time. Just apply it to the painful area, and then follow up with heat to help relax the muscles.

Lobelia

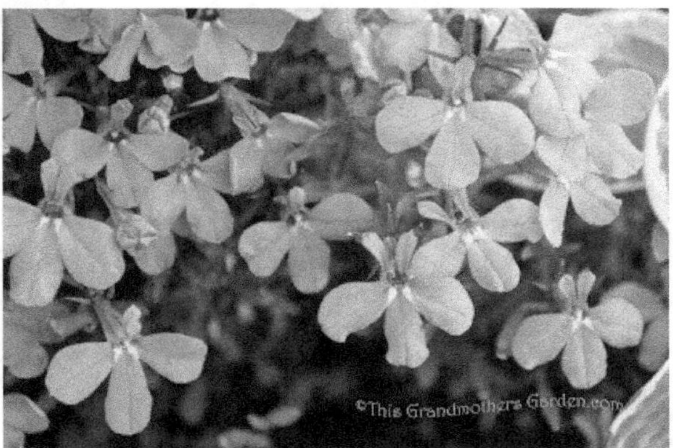

This herb is commonly used to treat asthma, but it can help with pain as well. It's best to use this herb in its supplement form so that you don't get the wrong dosage. Lobelia is toxic in high doses, so you should always be careful when using it, and it's best to have a holistic doctor to help you. This can be used in a tea, capsule, tincture, or as a dried herb. It has a mild sedative effect, and it works great for muscle and nerve pain.

Milk Thistle

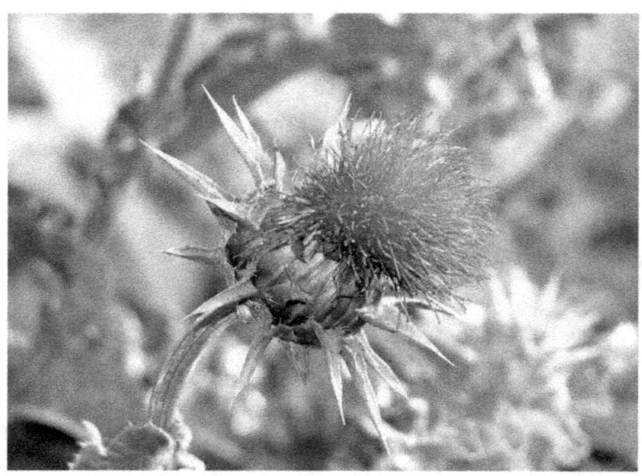

Milk thistle is known as a restorative herb, but it can also help with hepatic pain and swelling. It has anti-inflammatory effects, and it's most commonly used in tea. It can also help reduce high cholesterol. When using milk thistle to help with pain relief, it's best not to use it on its own. It's usually used with other anti-inflammatory herbs to provide long term relief.

Kratom

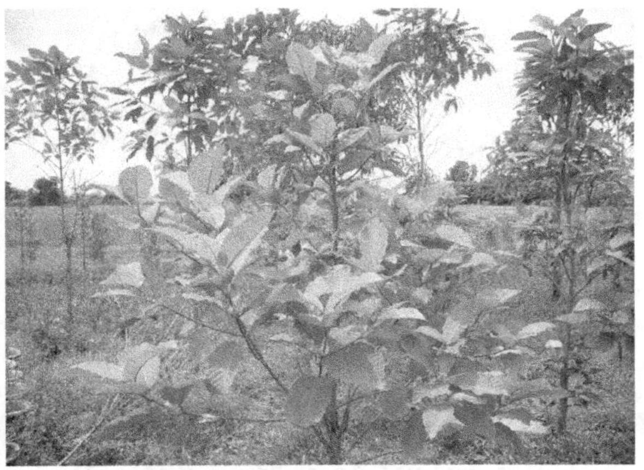

Kratom is a strong pain killer that will help while you're recovering, but it can be used for chronic pain as well. There are three types of kratom. The red vein variety is considered the strongest, and it will help to relax you and tense muscles that may be causing pain.

The white vein variety not only helps with pain, but it's also an antidepressant. The green vein kratom is a blend of the other two, but it's a milder vein for milder pain. Make sure that you talk to a doctor to make sure that this is right for you before taking kratom. You should not just add it to your daily routine.

Also it must be noted as of this time of writing, that Kratom is illegal in many countries around the world, or highly regulated. In the United States, several states and a few counties in states have made it illegal or have strong regulations. Be sure to check laws and regulations before purchasing.

Marshmallow Leaf

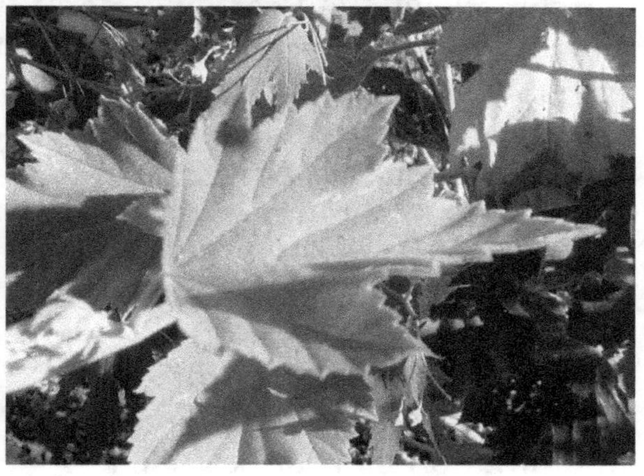

When people think of marshmallows they certainly don't think about pain relief. You're probably thinking about that fluffy treat that most people love, especially when it comes to s'mores, but marshmallow leaf can actually be a great pain reliever. The root is also known to help with pain. It is used for painful swelling, especially of the respiratory tract. It can also treat couch, inflammation of your stomach, stomach ulcers, and diarrhea. Marshmallow leaf can even be applied topically for insect bites. It can help with painfully chapped skin too. This is a pain relieving herb that is commonly used in conjunction with another to help boost pain relieving effects.

Passionflower

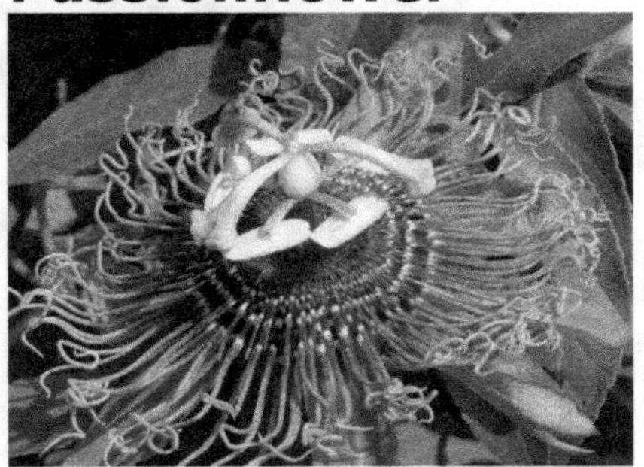

Passionflower is an antispasmodic, and it has sedative effects. It can work as a natural solution for your muscle pain, but it can also help with both tension headaches and premenstrual cramps. There chemicals in this flower to help both joint soreness and muscle spasms. It is easiest to find passion flower tea already made, but you can use a teaspoon of dried passion flower in a cup of hot water to make your own tea as well.

Burdock Root

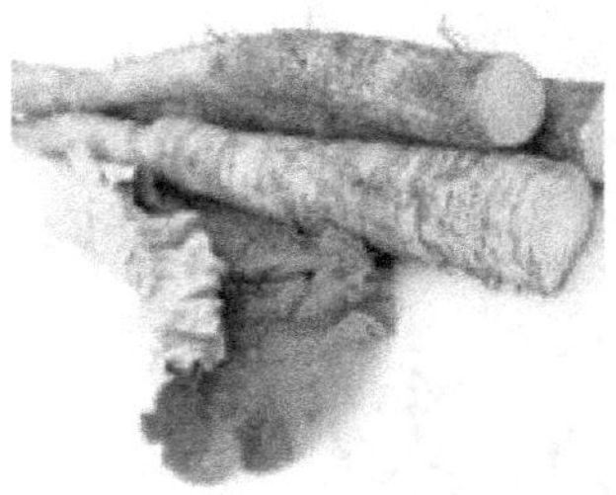

If you're suffering from arthritis pain, you'll want to increase your intake of essential fatty acids. Burdock root has a lot of fatty oils which will help you as well as it being an anti-inflammatory. You can actually eat burdock root in stir-fry, but some people will use the dried root as an alternative. You can make a tea by oiling it in water, allowing it to simmer for ten minutes, and then strain it. You can drink it warm or cold. Though, other people prefer to take this herb in capsule form, which the dosage will depend on your weight.

Nettles

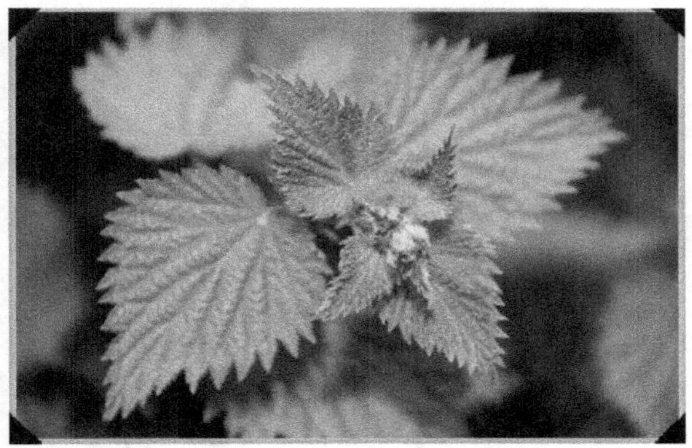

Nettles is a versatile herb, and it contains calcium, iron, magnesium, beta-carotenes, vitamin A, C, D, and B complex. It also contains calcium and protein. It'll help with pain from arthritis as well as gout, and it can ease pain while still helping to build strong bones. The most common way to use nettles for pain is through a tea, but it can also be used in a salve to help with arthritis pain when applied topically.

A Final Note

You can take many herbal remedies for pain by themselves, but they always work better when they're paired with other treatment. Of course, you should never add an herbal remedy to your daily routine until you've talked to your doctor to see if it works with your condition, any other medications you are on, or to simply see if it's regulated in your area. Changing your diet and working in foods that help to relieve pain naturally will make using herbal remedies more effective for chronic pain. There is no reason to just take one thing or just do one thing to manage your pain naturally.

Chapter 3: Supplements for Pain Relief

There are some supplements that can help you to get through and ease chronic pain as well. They're easy to find at your local grocery store or supplement store. Amazon has a market for them as well, making them even easier to find online if you're looking for a competitive price. Just remember to always talk to your doctor before you add any supplements into your daily routine, especially if you are on other medication.

Magnesium

This is a supplement that helps to curb pain, but you have to take it regularly. Though, you can also find it in pumpkin seeds and sunflower seeds. However, most people don't eat these often enough to get the magnesium they need to curb muscle spasms, pain from fibromyalgia or help to ease migraines.

Bromelain

This is another supplement that can help with stopping the hormone prostaglandins, which will reduce inflammation and pain. It comes from pineapple stems, and it's an enzyme you can find in the supplement section of your grocery store. It's effective in treating arthritis pain and other conditions associated with musculoskeletal tension. It can also help with trauma related inflammation, which will promote healing in both your connective tissue and muscles.

Vitamin D

If you experience frequent spasms or muscle pain, it's commonly due to a deficiency in Vitamin D. you can ask your doctor to check for this deficiency, and you can find vitamin D as a common supplement. Though, you can also find it in liquids or in your food such as eggs and milk. You should probably increase your exposure to sunlight as well if you have a deficiency, but this normally will not do enough on its own to correct the problem.

Fish Oil

You can actually cook with fish oil, but many people prefer to make a fish oil supplement if they don't like the taste. Fish oil can work as a natural pain reliever because it can block the production of chemicals such as cytokines and leukotrienes which are responsible for painful conditions such as psoriasis, gout, rheumatoid arthritis and inflammation. It also has omega 3 fatty acid which is known to treat lower black pain, neck pain, and menstrual pain. It can even help prevent the damage of cartilage which can lead to rheumatoid arthritis.

Chapter 4: Foods to Help with Pain

Your diet does matter when you are battling illness, but just adding in a salad once in a while or even adding kale to your diet isn't the way to go when fighting chronic pain. Most diets focus on detoxing or weight loss, but there are studies that show that food and ingredients in your food can help to relieve pain as well. In this chapter we're going to focus on foods that are known to help your body fight through pain.

Cloves

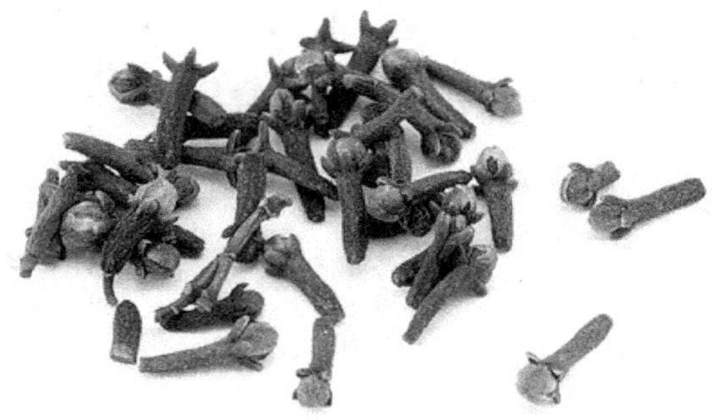

This is a traditional spice that many people will use for baking, but it's also been historically used for toothaches. It has analgesic and antibacterial properties. It has a compound called eugenol which will help to numb the area. Clove oil is commonly used, but you can use ground clove in many herbal remedies too.

Ginger

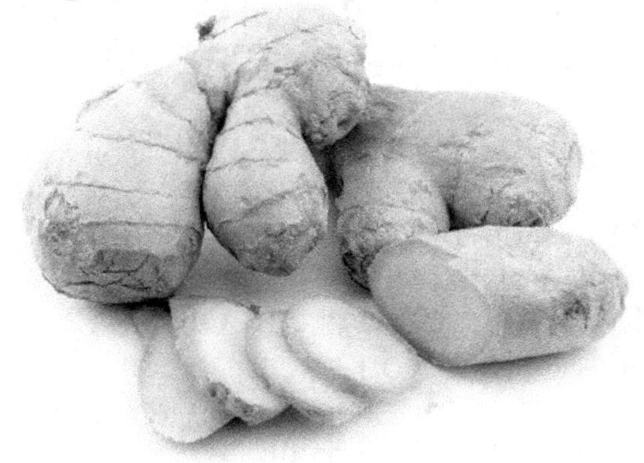

This is another spice that has many benefits regarding pain if you start cooking with it. It's well known for calming stomach pains, and it can block certain receptors to the brain which cause you to vomit. It can also help with chronic joint pain, inflammation, migraines and standard headaches, pain resulting from the flu or a cold, and pain from arthritis. If you don't want to cook with ginger, you can get it in supplement form too.

There is of course ginger ale, but you should avoid sodas due to the high sugar content. You can use ginger in juices, teas and smoothies as well as adding it to a variety of dishes. There are many Asian and non-Asian recipes that allow you to get a large intake of ginger. Though, it can take seven days before you see signs of ginger working. Ginger is a long term solution for your pain.

Yogurt

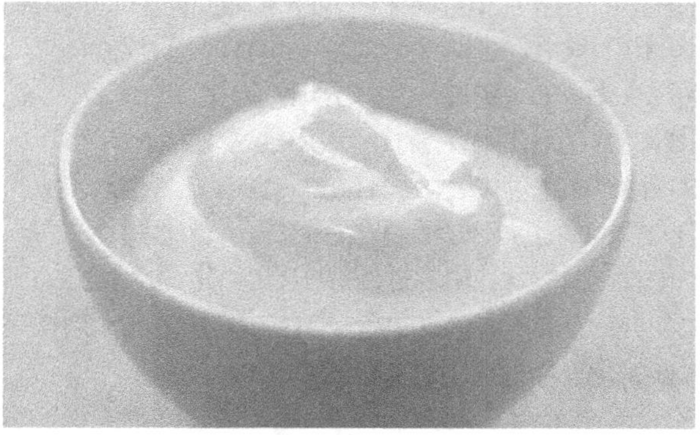

You already known that yogurt is great for your digestive system. Though, may people don't know that it can help with pain relief too? The same bacterial strains that help you get rid of bloating can help to attack what's causing your pain too. It's another great way to get rid of inflammation, making it perfect for helping with the pain associated with fibromyalgia. You just need to ingest it on a regular basis. Get the yogurt that says it has active live cultures. If you aren't getting the right yogurt, then it isn't going to work. Keep in mind that cheaper yogurts usually will lack active cultures.

Capsaicin

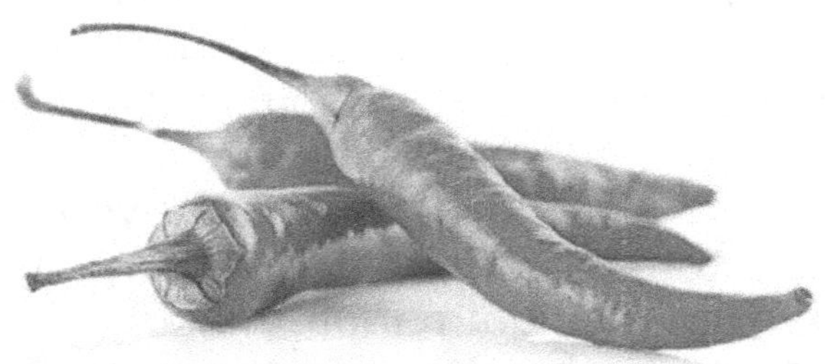

This isn't a food so much as it is an ingredient found in food. This ingredient is found in peppers to be exact. If you don't want to make too many diet changes or can't handle spice well, you can purchase capsaicin in its herbal form too.

This can work better than when you just add more peppers to your diet, and it can also be used topically this way. Capsaicin can be found in chili peppers, but it can also be found in cayenne peppers, jalapeno peppers and even bell peppers. It has almost no side effects unless you are sensitive to hot food or have an allergy to peppers. Capsaicin has been proven to help with a variety of pain by attacking and thinning out a substance known as P. this substance alerts your body to pain that you're experiencing. Capsaicin is especially important for muscle pain, but it can also help with headaches, lower back pain, PMS pain and joint pain.

Green Tea

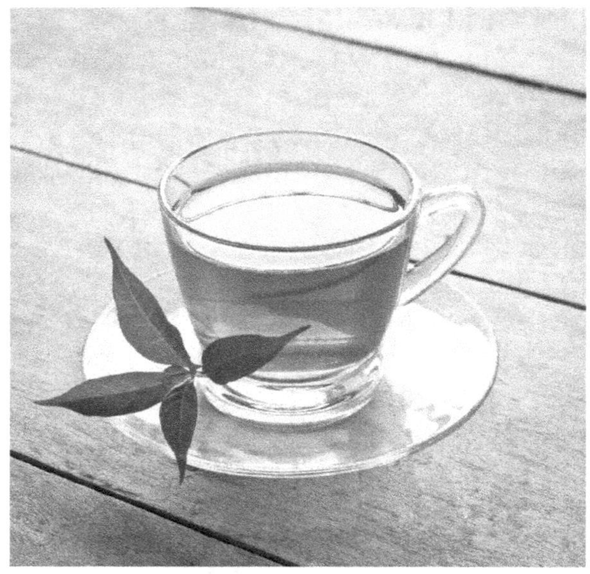

Green tea is great at helping with pain if it has to do with muscles, especially stiffness. It can be used with other herbal remedies to make them more potent to. Green tea has a compound that helps to relax your muscles, and the most common way to take it is in its tea form. However, you can also purchase green tea extract if you simply don't like the flavor or don't have the time.

Blueberries

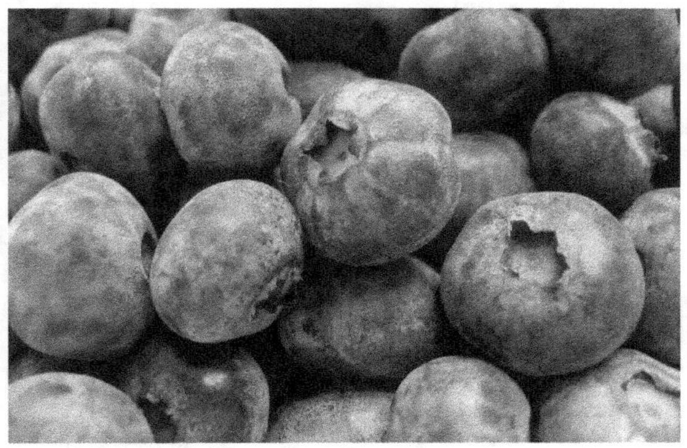

Most people already know that blueberries are full of antioxidants as well as anti-inflammatory properties. They can help repair your muscles too! There have even been studies that show that if you drink a blueberry smoothie both before and after an intense exercise you can avoid muscle damage. If you are suffering from muscle pain, adding more blueberries in your diet can help you to heal faster.

Cherries

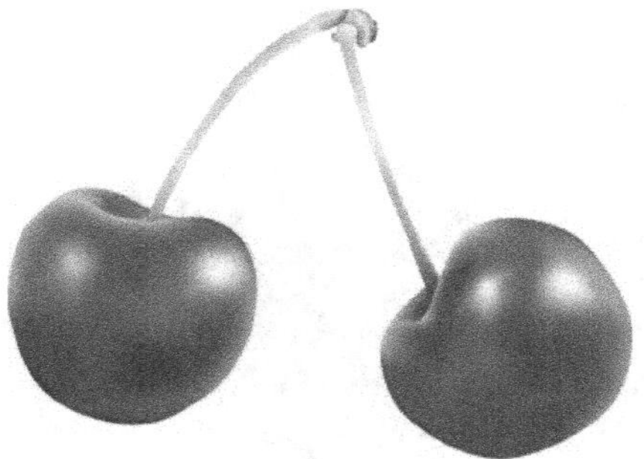

This is a food that many people have no problem adding into their diet to help fight pain. They can help with chronic pain issue because of anthocyanins, which is the same compound that turns them red.

They are also nutrient and antioxidant dense which will help your immune system to fight off inflammation in the long run. Anthocyanins will work on your brain in the same way that compounds in aspirin and Aleve do. If you don't want to eat fresh cherries, you can always drink fresh cherry juice too.

Peppermint

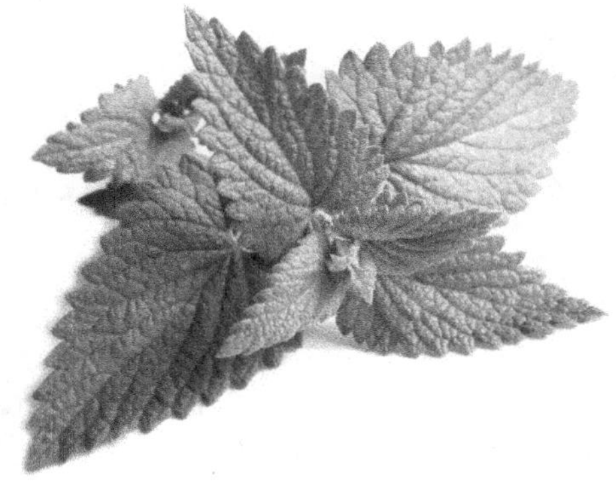

Peppermint is a great natural remedy for mild pain such as gas, bloating, joint conditions, skin irritations and toothaches. Peppermint extract can be applied to the tooth or gum to help with toothaches. You can also apply it topically in salves to help with various muscle pain. Peppermint essential oil can be applied at the temples or under the nose to help with headaches and muscle pain. Peppermint tea can be taken to help with more chronic pain. You can even add peppermint leaves to smoothies!

Licorice Root

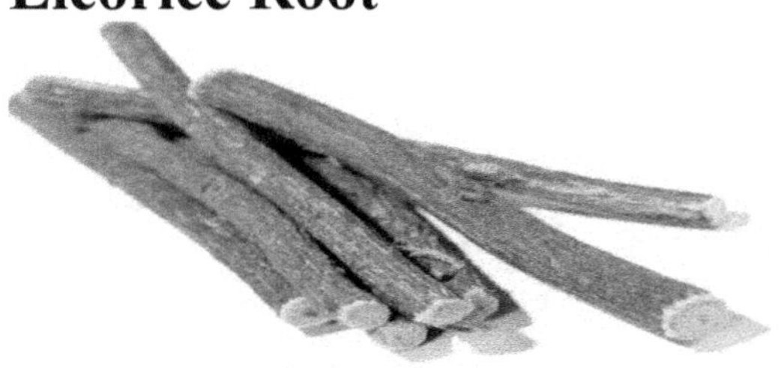

Licorice actually acts like corticosteroids, which is something your body makes to reduce inflammation. It will help to inhibit the enzyme production which will cause the inflammation process. It'll also help your body to release cortisol which will suppress your immune system, and ease pain that occurs with arthritis. If overdone, you can have issues with adrenal fatigue and anxiety, but it can be used safely in supplement form or as a tea if you use it carefully. You should not use licorice root if you have blood pressure issues. You should also avoid it if you have low potassium, heart or kidney disease.

Turmeric

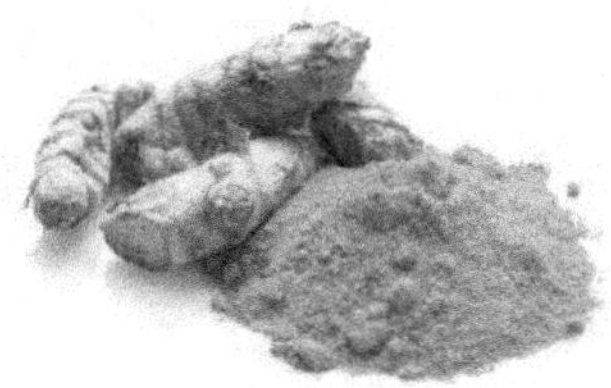

This is another ingredient, but you can find it as a spice too. Turmeric is mostly known for helping to fight back pain, especially if you are suffering from it long term. It can help with swelling, back pain, muscle pain and joint pain. Curcumin is a compound that can be found in turmeric, and it has anti-inflammatory properties. If you don't want to try to figure out how to add turmeric into your cooking, you can always use a turmeric tea which is easy to make as well as relatively cheap this will allow you to enjoy the benefits without trying to prepare a meal around it. If you want to make your own turmeric tea you'll need the following:

- 1 Teaspoon Honey, Raw

- Almond Milk
- ¼ Teaspoon Nutmeg
- ¼ Teaspoon Cinnamon
- 1/8 Teaspoon Clove
- 1/8 Teaspoon Black Pepper
- 8 Ounces Water

It's easy to make. All you need to do is combine your herbs and place them in your water. Let it simmer for fifteen minutes before straining your herbs out, adding in your milk and honey to preference. If you're in a hurry you can take boiling water, add in your herbs and blend so you don't have to strain. Just be careful when blending because steam can cause your blender to pop and explode if you aren't careful of the pressure. You won't need to strain if you're using a blender, and then you just add milk and honey to taste. If you notice that your stomach starts to become upset when using turmeric, you'll want to cut back on the dosage. Higher doses of turmeric do cause digestive tract discomfort in some people.

Chapter 5: Essential Oils for Pain Relief

When people think natural, they often think essential oils. Though, it's not always something people think about when they think pain relief. You can get natural pain relief using essential oils, and some of the oils can even be used on their own. Others you'll find work best if you pair them with other herbs or oils.

Lavender

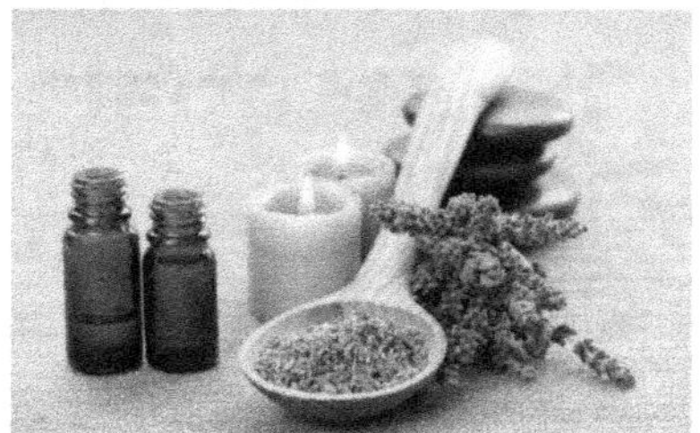

Many people think of relaxation when they think of lavender. Though, it can also be used to help with tension headaches and migraines. It can help you to sleep since it can cause a mildly sedative effect. Lavender is also an anti-inflammatory and an analgesic. You can use it to relieve sore muscles and general body aches by applying a few drops with a carrier oil such as coconut oil before rubbing it gently into the affected area.

Sandalwood

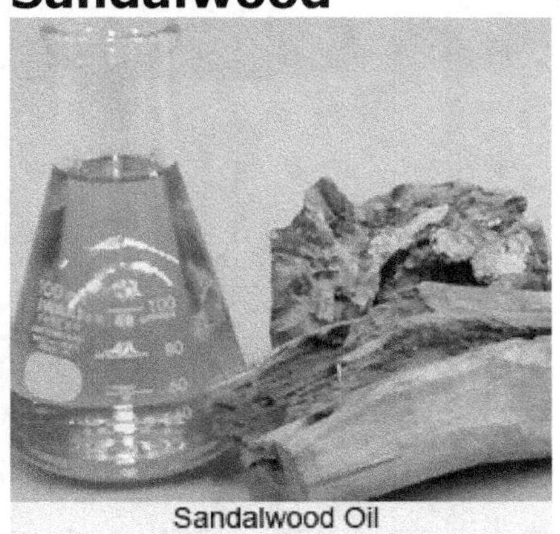

Sandalwood Oil

Sandalwood is an antispasmodic as well as an anti-inflammatory. It can help with skeletal pain, neuralgia, and even muscle pain. You can use a few drops in an infuser or it can be used externally in a salve.

Clary Sage

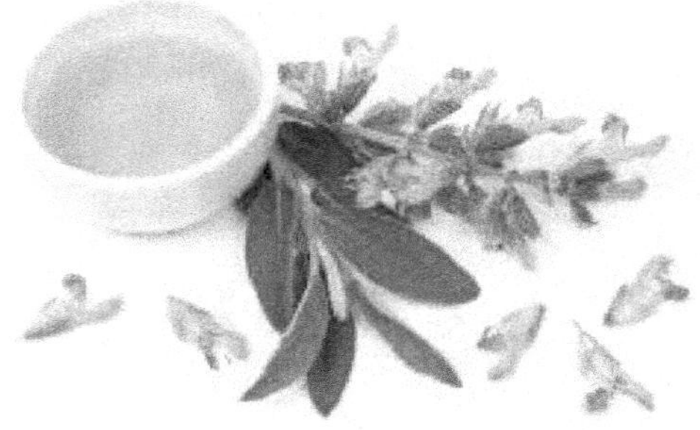

This essential oil helps with the pan
associated with menstruation and
menopause. It will also help with
stress induced headaches when
used in a diffuser. It can help with
painful stomach spams and cramps
when applied topically to the
abdominal area using a carrier oil.

Rosemary

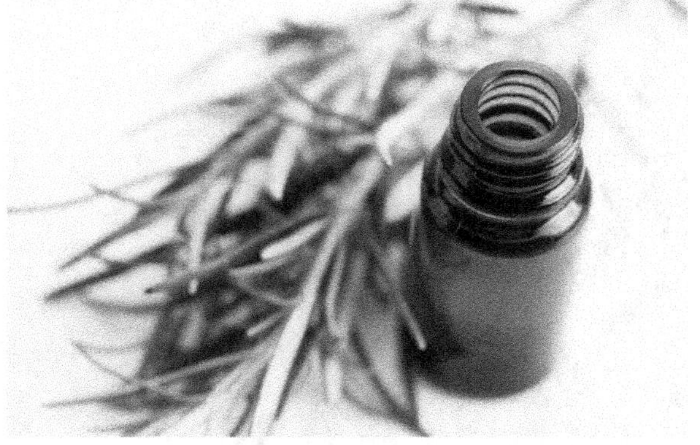

This is actually extracted from the culinary herb, and it's a powerful analgesic and anti-inflammatory. You can apply it topically for joint pain as well as muscle soreness, but it is not usually used on its own.

Pine

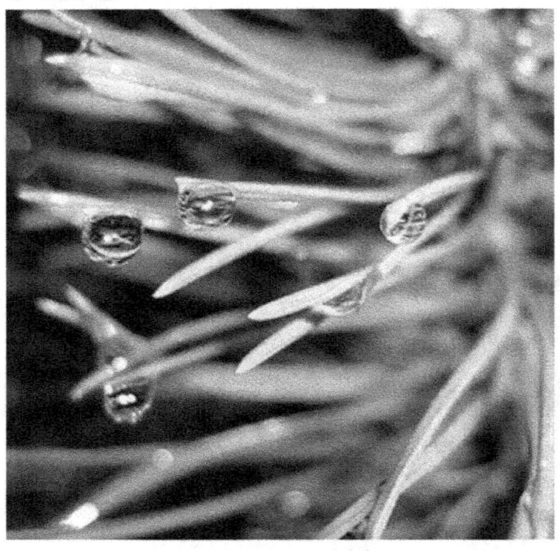

Pine is a great natural pain reliever for aches, general pains, sore muscles and even arthritis. It's often used with eucalyptus and peppermint essential oil for the best results. It will help to increase your circulation, which can help with joint pain as well. For pain relief, pine is commonly used topically with a carrier oil.

Marjoram

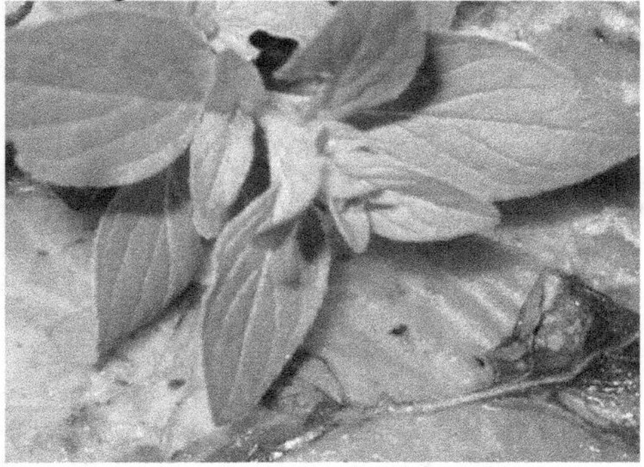

This can relieve muscular spasms from overexertion, which makes it great for short term pain. It can also be used for toothache. It has a sedative effect, which can bring relief from chronic pain, especially when dealing with osteoarthritis and rheumatism.

Evening Primrose

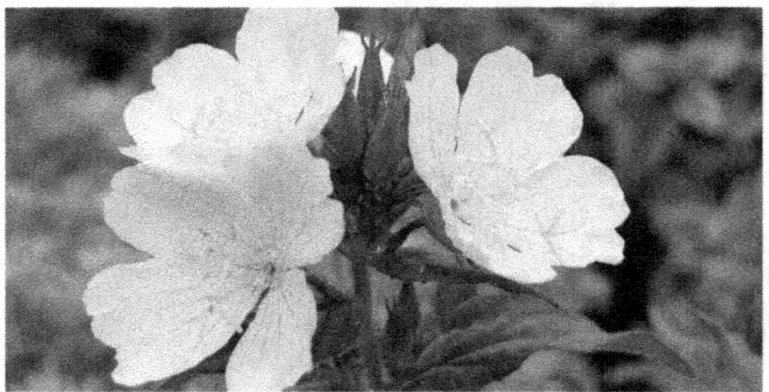

This is commonly used for skin conditions such as eczema, but it can also be used for pain such as rheumatoid arthritis. It has anti-inflammatory properties, and it is best used when used alongside a fish oil supplement.

Chamomile

Chamomile is another essential oil that most people think is only best for calming you down and helping you to sleep. Though, it can also help with headaches and has analgesic properties. Both German chamomile and roman chamomile can help with joint and muscle pains. Roman chamomile is milder and can help with abdominal discomfort. German chamomile is more effect if you're treating pain that is caused by an inflammatory condition. It's best for treating lower back pain as well as PMS related pain.

Eucalyptus

You already know that eucalyptus can help in its herbal form, but you can use eucalyptus essential oil if you find it easier to keep on hand. This can help with muscle pain, and it's an anti-inflammatory. Like any essential oil, you'll need to add it to a carrier oil before applying to your skin.

Wintergreen

This essential oil comes from North America, and Native Americans used it extensively since ancient times. Though, it's limited to external use due to toxicity. It's great at treating neuralgia and skeletal pains. It's commonly used to help with arthritis, sports injuries, and muscle pain. It can also help to relieve a headache when added to a headache balm.

Peppermint

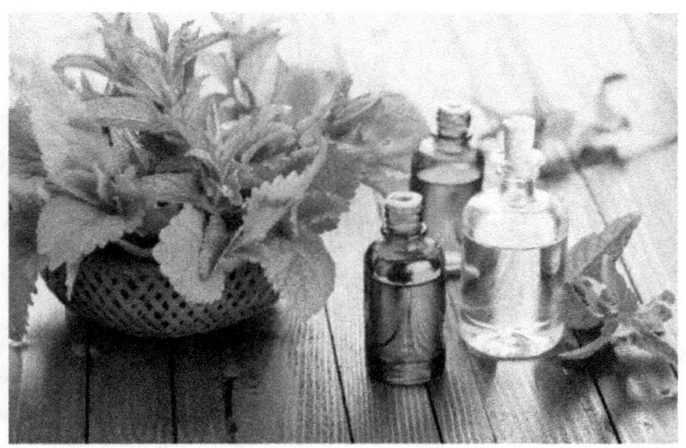

Peppermint essential oil doesn't just perk you up. It's also an antispasmodic, which can help with stomachaches, indigestion and nausea if you have a food grad essential oil. You can add a drop or two to water. You can use it topically to help relax your lower back, and it can reduce tension and pain caused by fibromyalgia as well as helping with headaches.

Chapter 6: Recipes for Pain Relief

In this chapter you'll learn some of the most common herbal recipes that you can use to kill pain naturally. There's no reason to use things on their own when you can get a better result if you pair them. Just remember that even these remedies will react to people differently, so it's important to keep track of which remedies do and do not work for you. This will help you to know what herbs commonly react to your body the way you need them to in order to manage your pain.

Leafy Relief

Once again you'll be using a tea as a base for this wonderful remedy. Feverfew can be grown fresh, and it will work better. Though, this recipe is for dried feverfew since it's easier to get ahold of. If you're using fresh feverfew, then just add a few sprigs and let steep for a few minutes longer.

Ingredients:
- 1 Teaspoon Feverfew
- 1 Teaspoon Black Tea Leaves
- 1 Teaspoon Ginger

Directions:
Tea:
1. For a tea, crush and roll your herbs in a paper towel before placing into your tea ball. Let them steep for five to ten minutes in warm water before removing and add honey to taste.
2. Drink twice daily or blend in a smoothie.

Salve:
1. Crush as small as you can, and mix into unscented lotion.
2. Apply to the affected area and leave on for about twenty to twenty-five minutes before removing gently with a warm, damp washcloth. You should repeat this two to three times daily.

Cayenne Salve

You already know how much putting capsaicin in your diet can help with pain, but you can make a topical cayenne salve to help with pain as well. It can be easier to use this salve rather than supplements if you aren't suffering from muscle pains regularly.

Ingredients:
- ½ Cup Olive Oil

- 2 Tablespoons Cayenne Powder
- ½ Ounce Beeswax, Grated

Directions:
1. You're going to want to infuse your oil by putting it in either a slow cooker or a double boiler. Make sure that it doesn't get hot enough to fry your herbal material. It's best if you can heat it to 0 degrees.
2. However, if you're using a double boiler you'll want to put one to two inches of water at the bottom. Put a tight fitting bowl on top. Place your oil and cayenne powder together, mixing and letting it simmer over medium heat for twenty minutes. The oil should be fairly warm.
3. Let it stand for twenty minutes, letting it cool off some.

4. Repeat this warming and cooling process for about two to three hours.
5. If you're using a crockpot, then keep it at 100 degrees for two to three hours.
6. Strain your infused oiler.
7. Heat your beeswax over low heat in a small saucepan, or you can use a double boiler, stirring until it's melted.
8. Once melted, add in your infused oil, and combine.
9. Pour into a tin or airtight jar, and let it cool.
10. Apply as necessary.

Invigorating Relief

This is great for chronic pain, but it can take up to two weeks before you see signs of relief. This is not a short term relief for pain.

Ingredients:
- 1 Teaspoon Ginger

- 1 Teaspoon Cinnamon
- 2 Teaspoon Turmeric

Directions:
Tea:

1. Mix like you normally would, crushing and placing in a paper towel in your tea ball. Let it steep for eight to fifteen minutes. The longer you let it steep in your warm water the better.
2. Add honey as desired, and take two to three times daily for maximum relief.

Salve:

1. Mix like you normally would after crushing into an unscented lotion and then apply.
2. Let sit for twenty minutes before wiping it away. It's best to repeat in the morning and at night.

Muscle Pain Cream

This cream is a little harder to make, but it will help with deep muscle aches. It can be used in the short term or the long term.

Ingredients:
- 2 parts Arnica Flower
- 1 Part Ginger Root
- 1 ½ Parts St. John's Wort
- 1 Part Comfrey Leaf
- 1 Part Peppermint Leaf
- ½ Part Cayenne Powder
- 3 Parts Olive Oil to 1 Part Coconut Oil
- ¼ Cup Beeswax

Directions:
1. Place your St. John's Wort, ginger, cayenne, comfrey, arnica and peppermint leaf in your carrier oils after mixing them together.
2. Heat at 100 degrees for two to three hours to infuse into your oil.
3. Use a cheesecloth to strain your herbs.

4. Let cool and heat your beeswax in a double boiler.
5. Mix in your oil, and then place in an airtight container.
6. Use topically as needed.

Simple Muscle Cream

This is another simple muscle cream that is highly effective, so that you don't have to wait around for relief.

Ingredients:
- 20 Drops Peppermint Essential Oil
- ¼ Teaspoon Ground Pepper
- ¼ Teaspoon Ground Ginger
- 20 Drops Eucalyptus Essential Oil
- 20 Drops Clove Essential Oil
- 1 Tablespoons Beeswax, Grated
- ¼ Cup Coconut Oil
- ¼ Cup Olive Oil

Directions:

1. Heat your oil up in a double boiler until thoroughly combined.
2. Mix well before melting in your beeswax.
3. Make sure it's mixed, and then take it off heat to add in your essential oils, ginger, and pepper.
4. Store in an airtight container, and use as necessary.

Versatile Healing

You can drink this as a tea or you can use the same ingredients to make a salve. The best part is that you only need three ingredients!

Ingredients:
- 1 Teaspoon St. John's Wort, Dried
- 1 Teaspoon Rose Petals, Dried
- 1 Teaspoon Capsaicin, Dried

Directions:

Tea:

1. If you're using it for a tea, then you'll want to crush the herbs and roll them in a paper towel or cheese cloth. Place them in a tea ball, and then soak in eight ounces of water. You should add a teaspoon of honey if it's too bitter for you. If you're working with powdered herbs, then you'll want to use the paper towel to make sure that the powder does not get in your drink.

Salve:

1. Crush your herbs as small as you can, and then mix with an unscented lotion.
2. Apply to the area that is hurting, and then take a warm washcloth to remove them after twenty minutes.
3. Repeat in the morning and at night as often as needed for comfort.

Green Tea Pain Killer

The base for this recipe is green tea, and so you'll naturally make it into a tea most often, but you can use it as a salve as well. Once again you're only working with three ingredient, so you won't have to spend too much to get the pain relief you deserve.

Ingredients:
- 1 Teaspoon Green Tea Leaves, Dried
- 1 Teaspoon Ginger
- 1 Teaspoon Cinnamon

Directions:
Tea:
1. Crush the herbs and then roll then in your paper towel before placing them in your tea ball, and then let it sit for five to ten minutes.
2. Add a tablespoon of honey as desired before drinking. It's best to drink two cups a day,

and you can blend it with fruit to make a smoothie too.

Salve:
1. Crush your herbs small, and then mix in with an unscented lotion. Apply to the affected area.
2. Let it sit for twenty minutes before removing with a warm wash cloth, repeating twice daily as needed.

Strong & Chronic Relief

Remember that you shouldn't use kava kava without talking to your doctor about it first. This is a stronger way to get rid of chronic pain, and it especially recommended for muscular pain.

Ingredients:
- 1 Teaspoon Ginseng
- 1 Teaspoon Kava Kava
- 1 Teaspoon Devil's Claw

Directions:
Tea:
1. Crush and then roll into a paper towel, placing in your tea through a tea ball. Let it steep for about ten minutes before adding honey to taste.
2. Do not drink more than two cups daily, and drinking one in the morning and one at night is recommended. It is also recommended to eat with this remedy.

Salve:
1. Just do as you normally would, mixing your crushed herbs into your unscented lotion and applying to the affected area.
2. Let it sit for about twenty minutes before removing with a damp wash cloth. Using it as a tea is recommended for overall pain, but a salve is better for pain that's concentrated in a single area.

Cramp Cream

Cramps are a legitimate form of pain, and if they are chronic it can start to wear on you. You'll find that this cramp cream will give you quick relief, helping you to get back to your regular routine. You'll find that this may be a little harder to make, but it's a strong cream that will last up to six months when stored properly.

Ingredients:
- 3 Ounces Arnica & Comfrey Infused Oil
- ½ Ounce Beeswax, Grated
- ½ Ounce Stearic Acid
- 1 ½ Ounce Shea Butter
- 1 ½ Ounces magnesium Oil
- 1 ½ Ounces Aloe Vera Gel
- 2 Teaspoons Aloe Vera Gel
- 2 Teaspoons Arrowroot Powder
- 5-6 Drops Lavender Essential Oil

- 5-6 Drops Peppermint Essential Oil

Directions:
1. Use a double boiler and melt your beeswax, herbal infused oil, and stearic acid in a jar.
2. Take it off heat and stir in your shea butter until melted. If you overheat your shea butter, then you'll have a grainy texture.
3. Let it cool, and then in another bowl add in your aloe vera and magnesium oil.
4. Warm together, but do not let it come to a boil.
5. Drizzle this mixture into your shea butter mixture, and then add in your arrowroot powder.
6. Whip together, and then whip in your essential oils.
7. Store in an airtight container and use as necessary.

Dandelion Salve

As promised, here is an easy DIY dandelion salve that you can make with fresh or dried dandelions. You can use fresh or dried dandelions in this easy salve recipe.

Ingredients:
- 15 Drops Lavender Essential Oil
- 1 Cup Dandelion, Fresh (1/2 Cup Dried)
- 2 Cups Olive Oil
- 2 Ounces Coconut Oil
- 2 Ounces Beeswax, Grated

Directions:
1. Start by infusing your olive oil with your dandelion by heating it at 100 degrees for three hours.
2. Strain out your dandelion, and let your infused oil cool.
3. Melt your beeswax and coconut oil together over a double boiler.
4. Slowly add in your infused oil, making sure to mix well.

5. Take it off of heat, and then add in your lavender oil.
6. Let it cool, and store in an airtight container. Use as needed.

Simple Pain Rub

It doesn't have to be hard to get relief from your pain, and you shouldn't have to always wait. This is an easy recipe to whip up whenever you need to.

Ingredients:
- 3 Drops Sandalwood Essential Oil
- 2 Drops Marjoram Essential Oil
- 5 Drops Wintergreen Essential Oil
- 3 Drops Lavender Essential Oil
- 2 Tablespoons Coconut Oil

Directions:

1. Just massage into the area, and you should notice pain relief within ten to fifteen minutes.

Nerve Pain Relief

This is a wonderful pain relief recipe that creates enough for a rollerball so that you can carry the remedy with you. There's no reason to let pain keep you from going where you want to.

Ingredients:
- 10 ml Roller Bottle
- 20 Drops Geranium Essential Oil
- 20 Drops Basil Essential Oil
- 20 Drops Lavender Essential Oil
- Fractionated Coconut Oil

Directions:
1. Add all of your essential oils into your roller bottle, and then fill with your coconut oil.

116

2. Shake before use, and apply
   to the area you're
   experiencing pain in.

Essential Oil Relief

This salve is completely made up of essential oils, and it's quick and easy to make. You'll be able to finish it within an hour, but to cool it down quickly place it in the fridge for five to ten minutes. This allows you to use the salve a little quicker.

Ingredients:
- 5 Drops Wintergreen Essential Oil
- 4-6 Drops Lavender Essential Oil
- 5 Drops Eucalyptus Essential Oil
- 7-10 Drops Peppermint Essential Oil
- 5 Drops Clove Essential Oil
- ½ Cup Coconut Oil

- 1 ½ Ounces Beeswax, Grated
- ¼ Cup Olive Oil

Directions:

1. Melt your beeswax in a double boiler with your oil, mixing together.
2. Take off of heat, and then add in essential oils. Make sure to stir well.
3. Store in an airtight container and apply as necessary.

Headache Balm

Ingredients:
- 6 Tablespoons Olive Oil
- ½ Ounce Beeswax
- 1 Tablespoon Magnesium Oil
- 20 Drops Peppermint Essential Oil
- 10 Drops Lavender Essential Oil
- 10 Drops Lemon Essential Oil

Directions:
1. Grate your beeswax, and
then place it and your olive
oil in a double boiler. Melt
and mix together gently.
2. Add in all of your essential
oils once you take it off heat,
and then place it in an
airtight container.
3. Rub on your temples as
needed.

Chapter 7: Pain Relieving Drinks

If you've tried turmeric tea, then you already know one pain relieving drink that will help you. There were options for teas in the chapter above, but this chapter will go more in depth with more complex teas and drinks that you can make to help with your pain. Some of these drinks can even be used daily to help with chronic pain, especially pain that is caused by inflammation.

Raspberry & Rosemary Lemonade

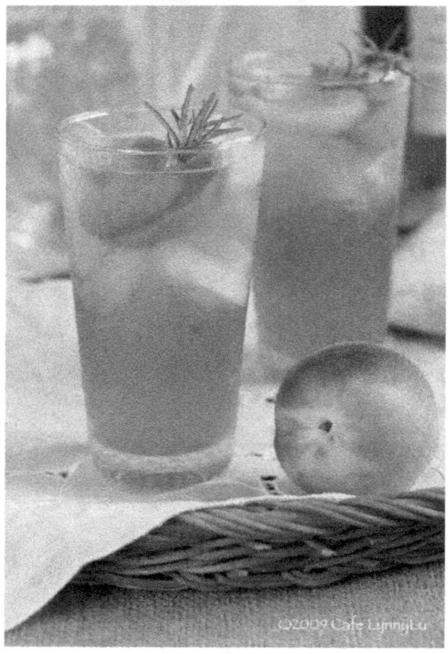

Not many people think lemonade when they think about something that can help with their pain. Though, it can actually reduce inflammation when you combine it with rosemary. This rosemary lemonade is a great way to up your rosemary intake on a regular basis, and it's full of antioxidants too!

Ingredients:

- 1 Quart Water
- 3 Lemons, Sliced
- ¼ Cup Rosemary Leaves, Fresh
- ¼ Cup Honey, Raw
- 1 Cup Raspberries, Whole
- Ice Cubes

Directions:

1. Start by oiling your water, and then steep your rosemary in it for teen to fifteen minutes.
2. Strain your rosemary out, and then stir in your honey.
3. Add in your other ingredients, and let sit for at least a half hour before serving.
4. Drink at least twice daily to see results.

Headache Lemonade

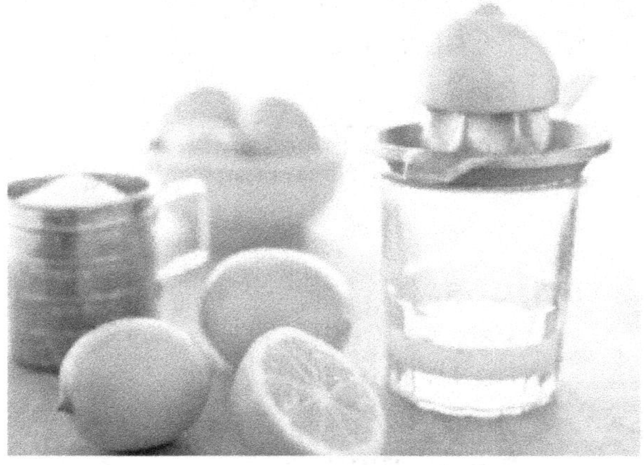

This headache friendly recipe will help with tension, stress, and inflammation headaches. It can also help to calm you down after a long day. You'll find that it can even help with stomach pain. Lavender will also help to lower blood pressure too!

Ingredients:

- 1 Cup Honey, Raw
- 12 Cups Water
- ¼ Cup Lavender, Fresh
- 6 Lemons, Juiced

Directions:

1. Start by boiling your water,
   and then add your lavender
   stalks.
2. Strain after letting steep for
   twenty minutes.
3. Mix in your honey, and then
   add in your lemon juice.
4. Make sure it's mixed well,
   and let cool before serving.
   Use as necessary.

Another Anti-inflammatory Smoothie

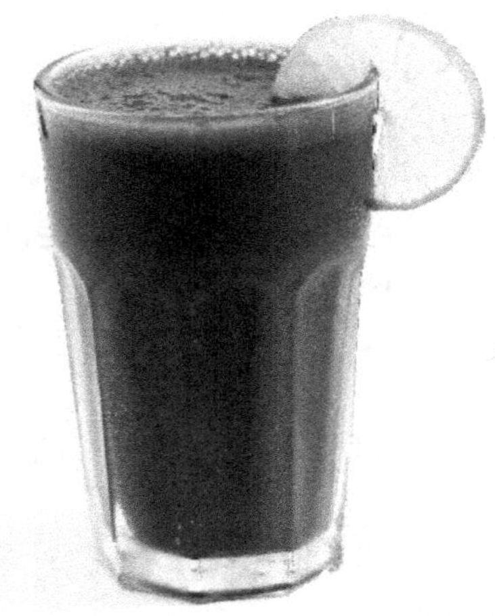

You already know how good cherry can be for both sore muscles and joint pain, making this a great anti-inflammatory smoothie that should be taken regularly for chronic pain.

Ingredients:
- ¼ Teaspoon Turmeric
- ½ Cup Blueberries, Frozen
- ½ Cup Cherries, Frozen
- ¼ Teaspoon Cinnamon
- 2 Cups Spinach, Shredded

- 1 Cup Almond Milk
- Ice Cubes as Needed
- 1 Teaspoon Honey, Raw

Directions:
1. Blend together until completely smoothie.

Turmeric Smoothie

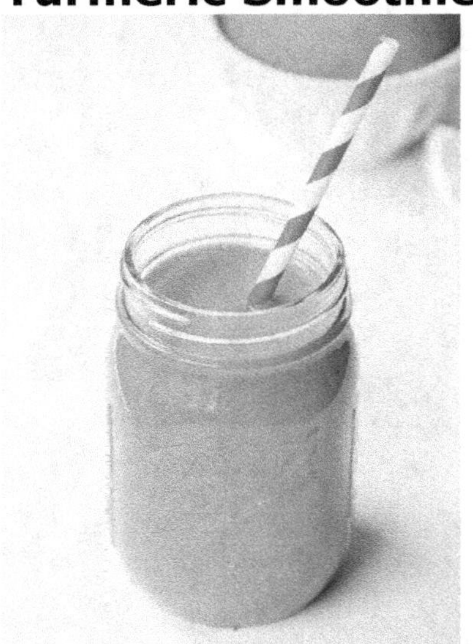

You know turmeric tea, but for some people it's a little too strong of a taste. Many people prefer this fruit packed turmeric smoothie instead.

Ingredients:
- 1 Cup Pineapple, Frozen
- 1 Cup Mango, Frozen
- 1-1 ½ Cups Water, Cold
- 1 Teaspoon Ginger, Peeled & Chopped
- 1 Teaspoon Turmeric Paste

- 1 Teaspoon Coconut Oil

Directions:
1. Blend all ingredients together until smooth. Add two tablespoons honey if desired.

Ginger Smoothie

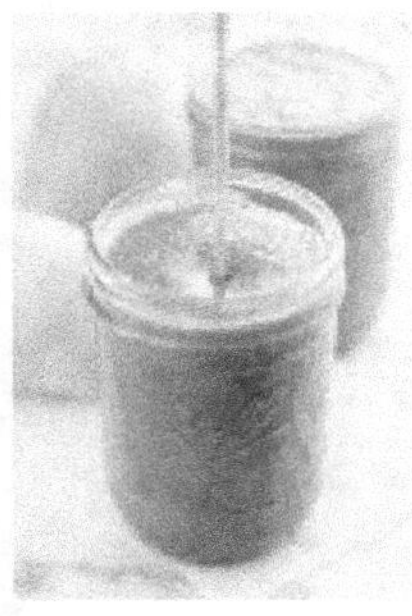

You already know everything that ginger can do for you, but it can be hard to remember to take a tablet each and every day. Some people even need more in their diet, especially at first, to see a difference. That's where this ginger smoothie comes to the rescue to help manage chronic pain.

Ingredients:
- 1 Banana, Frozen
- 1 Inch Ginger, Grated & Peeled
- ½ Teaspoon Cinnamon
- 1 Cup Coconut Milk
- 1 Tablespoon Honey, Raw

Directions:
1. Blend all ingredients together, and add ice if you want it to be thicker.

Back Pain Smoothie

Ingredients:
- 1 Teaspoon Ginseng
- 1 ½ Cups Green Tea, Cold
- 1 Teaspoon Honey, Raw
- ½ Cup Blueberries, Frozen

Directions:
1. Blend all of your ingredients in your blender, and add ice if you want to thicken it.

Arthritis Smoothie

This smoothie is great for arthritis, but it can help with almost any joint pain. Just remember that you won't see results right away. When you're dealing with natural pain relief, you have to be patient and continue with what works best with your body.

Ingredients:
- 2 Celery Ribs
- 1 Cup Grapes, Frozen
- 5 Basil Leaves, Fresh
- 4 Mint Leaves, Fresh
- ½ Cup Water, Chilled
- 1 Teaspoon Honey, Raw

Directions:
1. Blend everything together, and drink once daily.

Chapter 8: Pain Relieving Baths

Many people know how rejuvenating a hot bath can be, and it can certainly help with pain. What most people don't know is there are ways to make a nice, relaxing bath even more effective in treating the pain that you're experiencing. Though, you'll find that bath recipes are often better for muscle pain rather than joint pain. These bath recipes can often treat headache pain too! Check out these wonderful pain relieving bath recipes, and remember that like any natural pain relief, some recipes will work better for certain people than others.

Bedtime Bath

This bedtime bath is great at relieving mental fatigue as well as back pain, and it'll help you to get to sleep too boot!

Ingredients:
- ½ Cup Epsom Salts
- 10 Drops Lavender Essential Oil
- 10 Drops Roman Chamomile Essential Oil

Directions:
1. Just mix into your bath before getting in.
2. Soak for at least twenty minutes to get the full effect.

Apple Cider Vinegar Soak

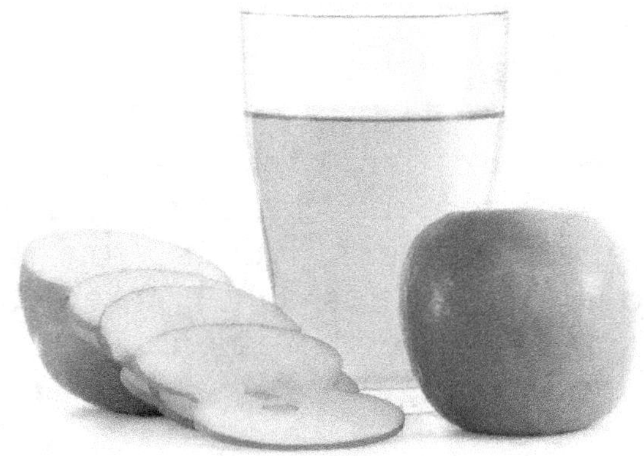

Don't let the name fool you! This common household ingredient is great to add to your bath for sore muscles, and if you rinse off there should be no lingering odor. However, make sure that you're using an apple cider vinegar that has the mother in it so that you get the full effects.

Ingredients:
1. ½ Cup Apple Cider Vinegar
2. ½ Cup Epsom Salts

Directions:
1. Stir in well before soaking for at least twenty minutes.

Essential Oil Soak

This is a great soak mixture to make for sore muscles. It can also help with mental fatigue, so you should not use this right before bed despite the lavender essential oil.

Ingredients:
- 3 Cups Epsom Salts
- 1 Tablespoon Sweet Almond Oil
- 4 Drops Lemongrass Essential Oil
- 3 Drops Lime Essential Oil
- 4 Drops Basil Essential Oil
- 4 Drops Lavender Essential Oil

Directions:
1. Mix together, and then add ½ of the mix to a bath to soak.
2. Soak for at least twenty minutes to get the full effect.

Comfortable Relief

This is a milder soak that will help you to get rid of daily aches and pains, especially after a hard workout. It can also help if you've recently pulled a muscle and are trying to recover.

Ingredients:
- ½ Cup Epsom Salts
- 4 Drops Peppermint Essential Oil
- 4 Drops Ginger Essential Oil
- 4 Drops Eucalyptus Essential Oil
- ¼ Cup Dried Chamomile

Directions:
1. Just mix into your bath and soak for at least twenty minutes.

Cinnamon & Lavender Soak

This is an odd bath recipe, but it'll not only smell nice but help you with your pain. It's known to relieve tension headaches as well as muscle pains and cramps.

Ingredients:
- 5 Drops Lavender Essential Oil
- ½ Teaspoon Cinnamon
- ½ Cup Epsom Salts

Directions:
1. Mix together and soak for at least twenty minutes.

Conclusion

You now have everything you need to help fight your pain naturally no matter if it's chronic or not. There's no reason to choose pain killers when you can dampen your pain naturally with less side effects. It even costs less, so start using natural remedies to help manage and reduce your pain. There's no reason to keep suffering when relief is at your fingertips. You don't have to plan your days around your pain any longer.

Lastly, if you enjoyed the book, cause you please take a moment to leave a review on Amazon? It would be highly appreciated!

Kathy Wyatt
www.FunHappyLives.com